Dr. Sebi

106

Approved Alkaline Herbs

How To Determine the Most Effective Alkaline Recipes To Prevent & Treat Different Diseases

Alkal Bassey

More of my beneficial informative Dr. Sebi's Therapeutic Alkaline Books for you are:

1. **Dr. Sebi Alkaline Diets Encyclopedia:** General Medicinal Alkaline Food Cell Diets and Herbs to Treat Various Diseases that Prevent Healthy Long Life Living

2. **Dr. Sebi** Secret Methods to Detoxify Body; Cure Cancer, Kidney and Liver Diseases, Prostatitis & Be Revitalized via Dr. Sebi's Alkaline Diets & Herbs

Table of Contents

Introduction

Why do you need the complete recipes of Dr. Sebi's approved therapeutic alkaline diets?

Dr. Sebi had greatly provided incredible formulations that had saved several sufferers from complicated health conditions like cancer, cardiac arrest, heart malfunction/diseases, kidney diseases, liver diseases, asthma, obesity, Human Immunodeffecient Virus (HIV), Inflammation, Arthritis, Eye defect, Erectile Dysfunction in men, infertility, Diabetes, High Blood Pressure…and many others that could not be cured by Western Treatments but managed with their conventional medicines till the sufferers ended up to untimely death.

Even though, there are some individuals disputing the methodology of Dr. Sebi's alkaline principles of treating different diseases that over a million sufferers had benefited from during his lifetime and after his demised.

Dr. Sebi believed in the philosophy of understanding the fundamental causes of any ailment, affected organs, body cleansing, detoxification and fortification with therapeutic diets that were completely provided in this Dr. Sebi 106 Approved Alkaline Diets.

For every cell of our body to effectively work well and performing self-healing against any danger from the bad intake of food containing high carbohydrate, refined fermented food or germs, we need to build a healthy internal environment that can only be achieved through diets made up of Alkaline medium.

Alkaline medium enables every cell in our body to perform awesomely, subsequently fight against all our health discomforts and rejuvenate body against aging.

6

Why diseases?

Truly, obesity is not what every healthy individual would desire for, due to the several health discomforts like high blood pressure, cardiovascular/heart diseases, self-unbearable overweight, fatigue, arthritis, joint pain, partial/permanent stroke, some prone to diabetes... and more others that are associated with the excessive unutilized fat deposit in the subcutaneous layer.

Many diseases are caused as a result of abnormal eating habits or eating unhealthy refined and fermented complex carbohydrate foods that engage the volume insulin for over 120 years to be exhausted within 20 years then Diabetes mellitus occurs; the food pH transform the internal body to become acidic environment that will hinder adequate metabolic reaction, enhances the rapid growth of any types of cancer (i.e. breast, prostate, skin, etc.) and cause more poor production of essential hormones like testosterone in men and progesterone in women which may lead to infertility, promotes acid-like bacterium(Helicobacter sp.) to cause ulcer; heartburn, dizziness, nerve malfunction, muscular cramp or inflammation, heart problems...and several others.

All these are what Dr. Sebi a competent naturopath and herbal practitioner put into consideration to formulate bio-mineral alkaline diets that could reverse and cure all the aforementioned health discomforts with a unique methodology that involve the understanding causes of the ailments, auto-regulation of the body with the observation of Fasting, Detoxing body system by neutralizing toxin (poison), cleansing approach through herbal medicine (cleanser) and revitalization of the body via his formulated medicine Alkaline diets and herbs that you will completely learn in this "Dr. Sebi Alkaline Diets Book"

During Dr. Sebi's lifetime, over a million of sufferers were benefited from his formulated Alkaline diets and herbal medicines that western treatment could not cure.

Chapter 1

What Makes Alkaline Essential For Your Health

There is a need for you to know why and how alkaline herbs, fruits, and extracts are very important to our health.

Naturally for us to live a healthy life, our internal body environment must be in a very good condition to enhance body homeostasis. The *homeo-* means a couple of things to work together in order to achieve a single pronounced result, while *-stasis* means for the result produced to be in a stable condition. Now, if you combine the words together *Homeostasis* you will have the stability of the internal environment of the body.

The internal environment of our body is made up of several essential elements which are also classified as micro and macro elements like *Potassium (K), Sodium (Na) Chlorine (Cl), Calcium (Ca), Magnesium (Mg), Nitrogen (N), Manganese, Selenium...many other; Organelle, Cell, Tissue, Organs and System and Fluid composed of large volume of Water and remaining volume is lipid.*

What is an Organelle?

An organelle is a minimum structure produced from the digestive essential nutrients such as Amino acids for proteins formation, phospholipid for cellular membrane, lipid for fat, steroid for hormone formation that determine the progressive formation of a Cell.

The collective function of various organelles in a cell determines the adequate function, viability, and survival of a cell.

For instance, in a computer system, there are many physical components called hardware. Inside of the individual Hardware, there are many components work together to ensure the function of singular hardware. Those smallest components that cannot stand on their own are the same as "Organelle" example of organelles are:

- Nucleus

- Ribosome

- Smooth Endometrium Reticulum

- Rough Endometrium Reticulum

- Golgi Body

- Lysosome

- Vacuole

- Chloroplast (Plant only)

- Peroxisome

What is a Cell?

A cell is a functional and structural unit exhibiting the general function of the living organism. When I mention a living organism, I mean living things which include we human, animal, plant, germs (i.e., Platyhelminthes, protozoan and bacteria). A cell could function on its own as an entity with the joint work of the organelles composed of. Example of a cell is *Somatic Cell, Stem Cell, and Germ Cell.*

What is Tissue?

A Tissue is the combination of cells working together to carry out a particular function. The examples of tissues are:

- Muscle Tissue

- Connective Tissue

- Epithelium Tissue

- Nervous Tissue

- Parenchyma (Plant only)

- Collenchyma (Plant only)

- Sclerenchyma (plant only)

- Xylem (Plant only)

- Phloem (Plant only)… and many others.

What is an Organ?

An Organ comprises two or more tissues working together to carrying out sequential functions in order to achieve a result. For instance Kidney, it has various tissues that carry out different activities to ensure that useful and healthy substances are not excreted with the by-product as a result, Bowman's capsule prevent the escape of blood into the Proximal Tubule and the epithelial layer of the tubule reabsorbs essential micronutrients and releases Urea and excessive salt into the urinary tract to be liberated with help of water. These are examples of Organ:

- Skin

- Heart

- Lungs

- Liver

- Kidney

- Root (Plant)

- Stem (Plant)

- Leaf (Plant)

What is a System?

This is when two or more or organs come together to perform a particular function in the body. It can also be called an Organ System. The examples of system are:

- Circulatory System (e.g., Heart, Blood Tissues and Blood)

- Endocrine System (e.g., Pituitary Gland, Pancreas, Thyroid, etc.)

- Excretory System (e.g., Kidney, Urinary Bladder, Ureters, etc.)

- Nervous System (e.g., Sensory Organ, Spinal Cord & Brain)

- Muscular System (e.g., Skeletal Muscles)

- Integumentary System (e.g., Skin & Hair, Skin Glands and Nails)

- Reproductive System (Testes, Ovaries, and Associated Organs)

- Respiratory System (Trachea, Lungs and other Associated Breathing Tubes)

- Skeletal System (Bones, Ligament, Cartilage, and Tendons).

- Immune & Lymphatic System (White Blood Cell, Lymph Nodes, Lymph Vessels, Bone Marrow, Thymus, and Spleen) {Campbell, Reece, et al. (2008)}

The survival of all the aforementioned level of general components of every living organism still solely depends on the concentration of alkaline solution revolving them.

If the body is appropriately kept in an adequate alkaline condition, it will facilitate the wellbeing of those organ systems of extreme importance in the body.

17

Alkaline medium enables all organelles to work very efficiently, enhances the reproduction of proteins for replacement of depleting enzymes, stem or somatic cells, hormones... and several others that perfectly determine the healthy living of every individual.

Alkaline prevents any abnormal occurrence or development of mild or chronic depressive illnesses in the body like cancer of any organ, Kidney inflammation, Liver defect, Respiratory difficulty, Internal bleeding, Arthritis, Diabetes, Ulceration... many others.

Therefore, the eating of foods having alkaline concentration will do you more help than you eating foods containing medium of acidity or the constituent of acidity suck as table sugar or synthetic product of sugar, alcohol, refined flour for bread, fried flour products their end result in the body increase the internal body environment to acidity, however, more of the foods that dangerous to our health according to Dr. Sebi will be comprehensively discussed in the next.

Acidity and Your health

It is no more a news that many of the synthetic and refined foods are extremely dangerous to our health due to the fact that, their end products in the our intracellular body fluid change body fluid pH level from alkalinity to acidity that can make all vital organ systems to be susceptible to poisons (systemic toxin), internal injury that can lead to bleeding, profuse tumor growth (Cancer), obesity, hypertension, partial/permanent stroke, diabetes, heartburn, arthritis, uterine fibroid…and several others.

What Are the Dangerous Diets to Avoid
1. Diary Meals

2. Wheat

3. Garlic

4. Fast Food

5. Seedless Fruits

6. Carboxylic Drinks

7. Alcoholic Drinks or Beverages

8. Candy and Can Foods

9. Yeast Containing-Diets

10. All Meats, Fishes or Eggs

11. Bread and Other Flour Products

12. Soy Bean or Soy Products.

13. Genetically Modified Organism

14. Sugar and Sugary Products

15. Superficial or Chemically Synthesized Flavor and Colorant.

16. Cranberries

17. Broccolis

Chapter 2

Curable Diseases with Dr. Sebi's Alkaline Diets List

First and foremost, there is a need for you to perfectly know those diseases you can use Dr. Sebi's Medicinal Food and herbs to cure and their cause. These are the various diseases Dr. Sebi cured during his lifetime.

- Pneumonia

- Cancer

- Sickle Cell Anemia

- Acquired Immune Deficiency Syndrome (AIDS)

- Leukemia

- Anemia

- Lupus

- Diabetes

- Arthritis

- Allergic Reaction

- Edema

- Liver Disease

- Eye Defects

Dr. Sebi's Healing Techniques

The healing techniques of Dr. Sebi are very unique and require serious self-discipline and determination. The mode of treatment is actually designed for a serious-minded and obedient individual that is ready to strictly adhere to every instruction and beneficial rules and regulations to ensure a perfect cure.

Dr. Sebi had been successfully practicing the natural alkaline therapeutic cells food for more than 30 years before his demise and there were numerous positive testimonies given by several sufferers of severe ailment that were completely cured.

Nutritional Precautions

In the *Nutritional Precaution* of Dr. Sedi, there is wonderful nutrition recommended for every individual to diligently follow.

1. The beneficiary must consume approximately 4 liters of Springwater in 24 hours.

2. Dr. Sebi's natural herbal medicine can be taken 60 minutes before any other medicine.

3. Constantly use Dr. Sebi's therapeutic diets without creating any break during consumption.

4. If you are accessible to where a few of the grains accepted by Dr. Sebi are produced in the dough, bread, cereal or pasta formation.

5. The potential curative effect of Dr. Sebi Diets sustains 2 weeks after the intake has been discontinued.

6. Prevent any meal prepare from Microwave.

7. Dr. Sebi Alkaline's curative formulations can be combined without any adverse effects.

8. Never consume any food, herb, fruit items not mentioned below.

The healthy diets are:

- Foods

- Fruit

- Vegetables

- Natural Herbal Teas

- Grains

- Nuts

- Seeds

- Oils

- Spices and Seasoning

  - Attractive Flower

  - Small Flavor

  - Spicy and Flavor

  - Flavors with Salt Sensation

Table 1. Healthy Organic Herbal Infusion

Common Name	Scientific Name
Chamomile	*Matricaria chamomilla* L.
Ginger	*Zingiber officinale* Roscoe
Tila or Sesamum	*Sesamum indicum* Linn
Burdock	*Artium lappa* L. *A.majus* Bernh
Fennel	*Foeniculum vulgare* Mill
Raspberry	*Rubus ideaeus*

Europe Elderberry or Black Elder	*Sambucus nigra* L.

Table 2. Healthy Organic Fruits

Common Name	Scientific Name
Moderate Size of Banana	*Musa sp.* L.
Ripe Pawpaw	*Carica papaya* L.
Sour Cherries	*Prunus cerssus* L.
Sweet Cherries	*P. avium* L.
Apple	*Malus domestica* L. Borkh
Tamarind	*Tamarindus indica* L
Corinthian Raisins Containing Seed	*Vitis vinifera* L.
Black Plums	*Vitex doniana*
Melons Containing Seed	*Cucurmis melo* L
Sweet Melon	*Cucurmis sp.*
Key Limes Containing Seed	*Citrus aurantifolia*
Prunes	*Prunus domestica* L.

Currants	*Ribes nigrum* L.
Grape Containing Seed	*Vitis vinifera* L.
Elderberry	*Sambucus nigra* L.
Figs	*Ficus carica* L.
Tender Jelly Coconut	*Coco nucifera* L.
West India or Latin Soursops	*Annona muricata*
Pear	*Pyrus communis* L.
Mango	*Mangifera indica* L.
Prickly Pear	*Opuntia sp.*
Tamarind	*Tamarrindus indica* L.
Sour Orange	*Citrus aurantium* L.

Berries in general, except Cranberries

Healthy Organic Vegetables

- Cucumber

- Mushroom Avoid Shitake

- Fresh Green Turnip

- Okra

28

- Garbanzo Beans

- Squash

- Mexican Squash Chayote

- Kale

- Zucchini

- Fresh Callaloo Green Amaranth

- Mexican Nopales

- Tamatilllo

- Olives

- Fresh Green Dandelion

- Fresh Cactus Leaves and Flower of Izote

- Watercress

- Bell Pepper

- Lettuce avoid Iceberg

- Verdolaga Purslane

- Fresh Dulse Sea Vegetable

- Avocado

- Fresh Wakame Sea Vegetable

- Fresh Nori Sea Vegetable

- Fresh Arame Sea Vegetable

- Onion

- Wild Arugula

- Tomato

Healthy Organic Grains

- Spelt

- Kamut

- Teff

- Amaranth

- Rye

- Quinoa

- Wild Rice

- Funio

Healthy Organic Nut

- Walnut

- Brazil Nuts

Healthy Organic Seed

- Hemp

- Fresh Sesame

- Butter of Tahini Fresh Sesame

Healthy Organic Oils

- Avocado

- Coconut avoid cook

- Olive avoid cook

- Sesame

- Seeds of Grape

- Hemp Seed

Dr. Sebi Super Healthy Natural Seasoning & Spices

Spicy Savors & Pungent	Moderate Savors	Sweet Sensational Savor	Salt Laden Savor
Savory	Bird Pepper of Africa	Purified Cactus Agave Syrup	Pulveriz ed Granulat ed Seaweed
Thyme & Dill	Fresh Cayenne	Date Sugar	Purified Sea Salt
Bay Leaves	Sage		Kelp
Sweet Basil & Basil	Achiote		Nori
Tarragon	Pulverized Onion		Dulse
Cloves	Habanero		
Oregano			

Chapter 3

Medicinal Benefits of Dr. Sebi Alkaline Diets and Herbs

The below therapeutic alkaline diets contain everything recipe you need in the formulation of healthy alkaline diets and its respective medicinal benefits that will enable you to be very sure of the healing effect of an alkaline food recipe you wanted to eat or prepare for a sufferer.

The general alkaline diets list will also restrict to determine your awesome health-promoting food and prevent you from eating or recommending correct items for others. It will also aid self-creativity, in combining the correct alkaline diets that could heal a particular disease. More so, you will be able to derive several delicious meals after fasting and remain healthy.

Common Name	Benefits
1 **Moderate Size of Banana**	Driving force of Nutrients, Rich in Potassium, Helps combats Anemia, Heart Health, Ease Digestion, Stabilize Blood Pressure.
2 **Ripe Pawpaw**	It helps in weight loss and improves the immune system. It helps the digestive system. It helps to fight diabetics. Help eye health. Protects against arthritis. It helps ease menstrual pain.

This plant assists in the treatment

3

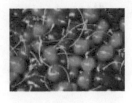

Sour Cherries

4

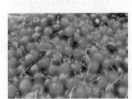

Sweet Cherries

of osteoarthritis, muscle pain, fibromyalgia, muscle soreness after exercise, diabetes, high blood pressure, gout, and insomnia.

This plant contains Antioxidant, anti-inflammatory, anti-cancer, cardiovascular properties.

5

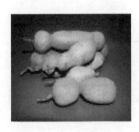

Tamarind

They are nutritious, help weight loss, help Heart health, help fight Diabetes, helps in the prevention of Cancer, and combat Asthma.

This plant fight against heart disease, cancer, diabetes, lower

6

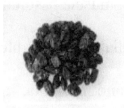

Raisins

blood sugar, lose bodyweight and

reverse fatty liver disease.

7

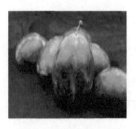

Black Plums

This plant helps fight constipation,

improves heart health, prevent

anemia, build strong bones,

improves teeth health, reduce the

risk of cancer.

8

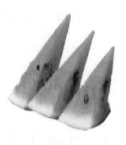

Melons with Seed

Helps the digestive system, assists

in weight loss helps oral health

and reduces

Cancer risk.

8 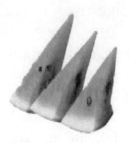 **Melons with seed**	Control blood sugar level, help in hair growth, prevent osteoporosis and contains potassium with other essential nutrients.
9 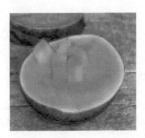 **Sweet Melon**	It contains nutrients, helps in the reduction of Blood Pressure level, helps Bone Health, stabilize Blood Sugar Control, rich in the electrolyte, improve Immune System.
10 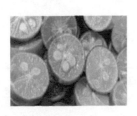 **Key Limes with Seeds**	Protect the skin, assist I hair growth, fight against cancer cells, prevent kidney stones, reduce inflammation…and many others

11	Improves digestive health, contains an increased amount of fiber, which helps prevent hemorrhoids, rich in potassium, rich in vitamins, rich in iron, improves bone health, reduces blood pressure levels and reduces cholesterol levels.

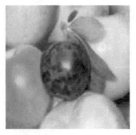

Prunes

12	It contains a rich amount of antioxidants and anthocyanins which help improves the immune system, soothe sore throats, and ease flu symptoms.

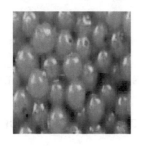

Currants

13	Controls blood pressure, helps in blood flow, decrease oxidative

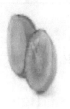

Grape with Seed

damage, help in the improvement of collagen levels and bone strength, fights cancer disease, helps in brain health, increase functions of the kidney, and prevents infectious growth. ...

14

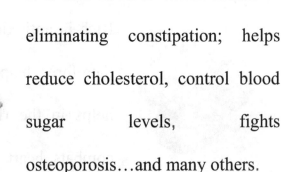

Figs

It is rich in fiber which assists in eliminating constipation; helps reduce cholesterol, control blood sugar levels, fights osteoporosis…and many others.

15

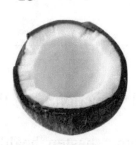

Tender Jelly

It contains an increased amount of fiber which helps in constipation, balances blood sugar level, reduces cholesterol…and many

Coconut	others.

16

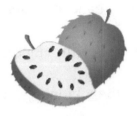

West India or Latin Soursops

Helps in fighting cancer, assists in weight loss, fight Gout, inflammation, and arthritis…and many others

17

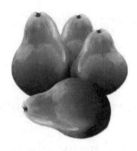

Pear

Rich in antioxidants, and fiber. It, therefore, helps in weight loss, helps in the risk of cancer, and combats heart diseases and fight against diabetes…and many others.

18

Provide good function of the digestive system, hasten healthy

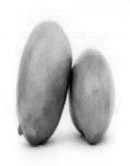

Mango

digestion, improves the health of the gut, helps in increasing weight loss, improves the health of the eyes, improves the immune system, reduces Cholesterol, helps fight Diabetics…and many others.

19

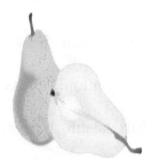

Prickly Pear

Rich in antioxidants, and fiber. It, therefore, helps in weight loss, helps in the risk of cancer, and combats heart diseases and fight against diabetes…and many others.

20

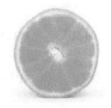

Sour Orange

Fights against angina, allergies, insomnia, nasal congestion, nerve pain, poor appetite, liver and

Types of Approved Berries You Can Eat

Do not eat **Cranberries.**

Berries	Nutritional and Medicinal Benefits
21 **Elderberry**	It contains a rich amount of antioxidants and vitamins which increase the immune system. It also helps reduce inflammation, stress, helps improves heart health, hinders and eases cold and flu.
22 **Raspberry**	It contains a reduced amount of calories, rich in fiber, vitamins, minerals, and antioxidants. They prevent diabetes, cancer, obesity,

arthritis…and many more.

23 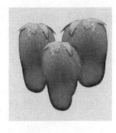 **Strawberry**	It contains vitamin C, Manganese and tender fiber that prevents constipation, heart diseases, inflammation, gets rid of oxidative tension, purifies the blood by removing bad cholesterol.
24 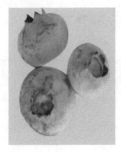 **Blueberry**	It contains Vitamin C, Vitamin K, Manganese, tender fiber, an antioxidant that suppresses oxidative stress, enhances insulin which in turn, prevents type 2 diabetes, improves memory alertness, retentiveness, and sense organ.
25	It contains Iron, Vitamin A, Vitamin C, Tender Fiber that prevent

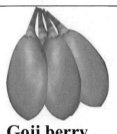 **Goji berry**	constipation. It improves clear vision; facilitates the removal of abnormal fat within the wait region and causes weight loss.
26 **Apples**	Antioxidant, weight loss, heart disease, type 2 diabetes, cancer, mouth sore, reduces bad LDL cholesterol. Prevents stroke, Vitamin a, b1, b2, b6, c, k, potassium,

Common Name	Benefits
27	Decrease menstrual pain, fight Diabetes reduces blood sugar level, fights against osteoporosis,

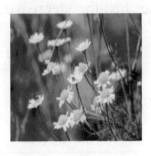

combats inflammation, prevents and fight cancer cells, helps in relaxing the muscles and fight cold…and many others.

Chamomile

28

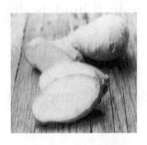

Ginger

It contains a compound called Gingerol, which is highly powerful to fight against infections. Helps for the treatment of Nausea, reduces muscle pain, fights osteoarthritis and soreness…and many more.

29

Rich in Fiber, reduce Cholesterol level, reduce Triglycerides level, stabilized Blood Pressure,

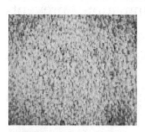

Tila or Sesamum

improves bone health, decrease inflammation and assists in forming cells...and many more.

30

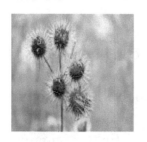

Burdock

Rich source of antioxidants, which helps in the removal of toxins in the blood. It hinders the multiplication of cancer cells, it increases libido and improves skin health.

31

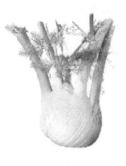

Fennel

Stabilized Blood Pressure, decrease the retention of water in the body, fights against Constipation, helps in fighting acne, Indigestion, Bloating, fights

Asthma, Purify the Blood, helps in eye health…and many others.

Healthy Organic Vegetables	Medicinal Benefits
32 Cucumber	Rich in antioxidants, helps in Hydration, helps in Weight Loss, and reduces Blood Sugar level. It contains several vitamins and minerals essential for the body.
33	It contains vitamin A which helps in Improving skin and hair. It reduces anemia, prevents Osteoporosis,

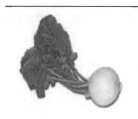

Fresh green Turnip

hinders cancer, fights against Diabetes, helps in

Easy digestion of food and facilitates conception…and many more.

34	It's rich in magnesium, folate, fiber, antioxidants, vitamin C, A, and K1. Assist women during conception; facilitate easy delivery in women, help heart health, blood sugar control and fight against cancer…and many more.

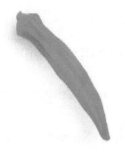

Okra

35	Rich in Plant-Based Protein, Controls Appetite, helps in weight loss, maintains Blood Sugar level

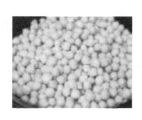

Garbanzo beans	and helps in easy digestion of food…and many others.
36 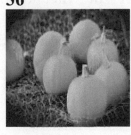 **Squash**	It is rich in vitamins A, B6, and C, folate, magnesium, fiber, riboflavin, phosphorus, and potassium…and many more.
37 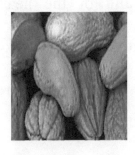 **Mexican Squash Chayote**	It contains a high content of nutrients and antioxidants. Improves heart health, balance blood sugar level, helps during conception, improves liver functions, fights against cancer, prolong aging…and many more.
38	This plant is rich in Antioxidants such as Quercetin and Kaempferol.

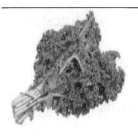 **Kale**	It contains Vitamin C and K. fights against Herpes virus, reduce cholesterol level in the blood, decrease the danger of heart attack…and many more.
39 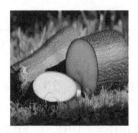 **Zucchini**	It contains a rich source of Vitamins C, A, potassium, folate, and fiber. Improve the health of the heart, reduce the danger of stroke, reducing high blood pressure, cholesterol
40 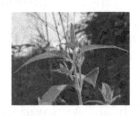 **Fresh Callaloo Green**	It contains calcium, magnesium, potassium, phosphorus, iron and vitamin C.

Amaranth

41	Contains Antiviral properties, antioxidant properties, stabilized blood sugar levels, fight prostatitis, decrease the level of cholesterol in the body…and many more.

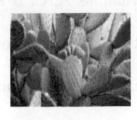

Mexican Nopales

42	Prevention of cancer, stabilize blood sugar level, improve vision…and many more.

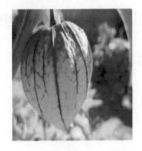

Tamatilllo

43	Contain antioxidants, improve heart health, prevents cancer, increase bone health…and many more.

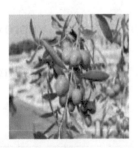

Olives

44  **Fresh Green Dandelion**	Rich source of vitamins A, C, B K, E, and folate. It also contains iron, calcium, magnesium, and potassium.
45 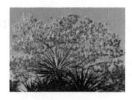 **Fresh Cactus Leaves and Flower of Izote**	Stabilize blood sugar, healing wounds, prevention of disease and reducing cholesterol.
46 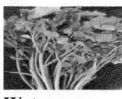 **Watercress**	Rich in Antioxidant fight against Diseases, prevent cancer, improve heart health, fight against Osteoporosis.

47 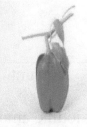 **Bell Pepper**	Rich antioxidants, vitamins C and carotenoids. They help eye health and decrease the dangers of chronic diseases.
48 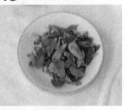 **Verdolaga Purslane**	Rich in antioxidants, omega-3 fatty acids, vitamins, and minerals. It helps in abnormal uterine bleeding, asthma, and diabetes.
49 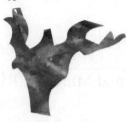 **Fresh Dulse Sea Vegetable**	It contains calcium and potassium which helps in improving bones, reduce blood pressure, improve your eyesight and improve the health of the thyroid gland.
50 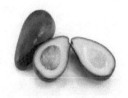	Rich in Potassium. It contains Monounsaturated Fatty Acids that promote heart health, reduce

Avocado	Cholesterol and Triglyceride Levels in the body.
51 **Fresh Wakame** **Sea Vegetable**	Contains the rich amount of nutrient, contain high iodine amount which helps the Thyroid gland, helps in weight loss, balance the blood pressure in the body, helps heart health, fight against cancer, improve insulin resistance and balance blood sugar level.
52 **Fresh Nori** **Sea Vegetable**	Rich in Vitamins and Minerals. Rich in Antioxidants. It is also rich in Tyrosine, Which Supports Thyroid Function. It improves gut health, decreases the

risk of heart disease, and reduce weight.

53 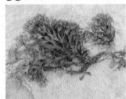 **Fresh Arame Sea Vegetable**	Rich in Vitamins and Minerals. Rich in Antioxidants.
54 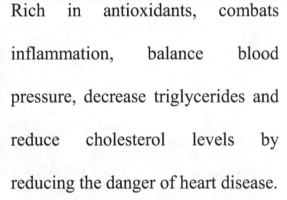 **Onion**	Rich in antioxidants, combats inflammation, balance blood pressure, decrease triglycerides and reduce cholesterol levels by reducing the danger of heart disease.
55 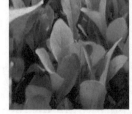	Rich in antioxidants, Calcium, potassium, vitamin C, B, and K. Facilitates blood to clotting, helps heart and nerve function, and

Wild Arugula	improves the body's immunity.
56 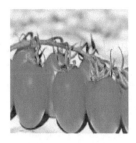 **Tomatoes**	Rich in the antioxidant lycopene, which helps in fighting many health conditions. Combats cancer, heart diseases. They are also rich in vitamin C and K, potassium, and folate.
57 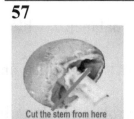 Cut the stem from here **Mushroom** **Avoid Shiitake**	It contains vitamin B and antioxidants which help to improve and balance the immune system. It also prevents damage to cells and tissues…and many others.

The advisable edible mushrooms you can eat after you have completed fasting. The recommended mushrooms have high potent of antioxidant, anti-carcinogenic, anti-inflammatory properties… and some essential nutritional benefits which I have mentioned in the table below. Please do not eat **Shiitake mushroom**

Approved Edible Mushrooms	Nutritional & Medicinal Benefit
57 Cut the stem from here **Portobello** *Agaricus bisporus*	It contains Potassium, Copper, Niacin, Pantothenic Acid, Vitamin B_2, and Selenium. It is an antioxidant, prevents inflammation within mucous lining…etc
58 **Porcini** *Boletus edulis*	It contains Iron, Sodium, Calcium, Potassium, Copper, Niacin, Pantothenic Acid, Vitamin B_2, and Selenium. Antioxidant, Anti-inflammation and strength muscular

tissues.

It reverses high blood pressure, reduces bad cholesterol, elevates HDL, and prevents heart diseases.

| 59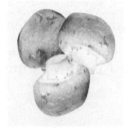
Cremini | It contains Phosphorus, Potassium, Copper, Niacin, Pantothenic Acid, Vitamin B_2, Vitamin C, Fiber and Selenium. It has Anticancer, Antioxidant, Treats Cardiovascular condition and regulates estrogen and other female reproductive hormones. |

| 60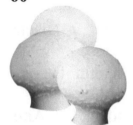
White Button | It contains Phosphorus, Potassium, Copper, Niacin, Pantothenic Acid, Vitamin B_2, and Selenium.

It enhances the general immune system and for supportive tissues |

(bone) and healthy brain

61 **Wild Morels** *Morchella*	It contains Zinc, Manganese, Iron, Phosphorus, Copper, Vitamin B_2, and Vitamin D, calms or prevents oxidative stress, anti-inflammation, anticancer, antioxidant, triggers immune-efficiency... etc.
62 **Enoki** *Flammulina velutipes*	It contains Potassium, Phosphorus, Niacin, Pantothenic Acid, Vitamin B_2, Thiamin, Folate, enhances the immune system, effective coordination of the nervous system, protects heart, reverses high blood pressure, fights against liver diseases, bad cholesterol, stomach illness.
	It contains Iron, Potassium,

63 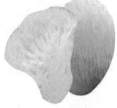 **Oyster**	Phosphorus, Niacin, Pantothenic Acid, Vitamin B_2 and Copper. Reduces triglycerides in the body, anti-inflammation, antioxidant, destroy and prevents the growth of cancer cells.
64 **Lion's Mane**	It prevents depression, dementia, anti-inflammation, antioxidant, heart diseases, ulceration, cancer, enhances immune system and diabetes.

Healthy Organic Nut	Benefits
65	It contains a rich amount of Antioxidants, Omega-3s. Reduces Inflammation, helps gut health,

Walnut	prevents cancer, stabilizes body weight, fights against blood pressure and diabetes.
66 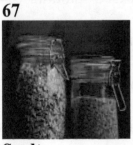 **Brazil Nuts**	It contains antioxidants, vitamins, minerals, and selenium. It reduces inflammation, supports brain function, improves your thyroid function and heart health.

Healthy Organic Grains	Benefits
67 **Spelt**	Rich in iron, magnesium, and zinc. Helps in heart health, aid digestion, reduce the danger of diabetes and stabilize the body weight.

68	It contains proteins, thiamin, iron, and zinc, fiber, vitamin E and calcium. It prevents constipation, improves cell growth, antioxidant, enzymes development, and no gluten.
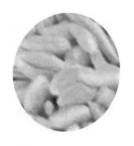 **Kamut**	
69	Contains Protein, dietary fiber, gluten absent, Magnesium, Vitamin B6, Zinc, Calcium, and Vitamin C. improves colon health, reduce blood sugar, and helps reduce weight.
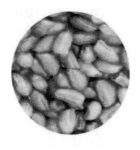 **Teff**	
70	It is a highly nutritious, gluten-free grain with an increased amount of fiber, protein, and micronutrients. It helps in lowering inflammation, cholesterol levels weight.
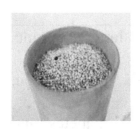 **Amaranth**	

71	Stabilize blood-sugar level, stabilize
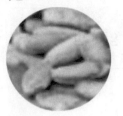 **Rye**	blood pressure level, improves heart health and helps in the reduction of cholesterol level in the body.
72	It contains a high amount of protein
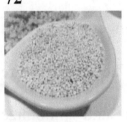 **Quinoa**	and fiber. It is also a rich source of lysine, magnesium, Riboflavin, and manganese.
73	It contains a rich amount of
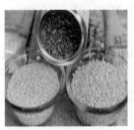 **Wild Rice**	antioxidants, protein, and other essential nutrients. It also recovers heart health and reduces the danger of diabetes in the body.
74	Helps in the following: heart health,
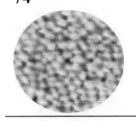	diabetes, digestion, weight loss, prevent anemia, detoxifying the body,

Fonio	gives Energy and contain no gluten.

Seeds	Medicinal Benefits
75 **Hemp**	Decreases the danger **of** Heart Disease, helps skin health, they are plant-based protein and minimize menopausal crises.
75 **Butter of Tahini Fresh Sesame**	It contains a rich amount of vitamins, and minerals, and antioxidants. Fight against some diseases in the body. It contains antibacterial and anti-inflammatory components. Fights against cancer disease, and helps kidney health.

Healthy Organic Oils	Benefits
76 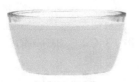 **Avocado oil**	Rich in Potassium. It contains Monounsaturated Fatty Acids that promote heart health, reduce Cholesterol and Triglyceride Levels in the body.
77 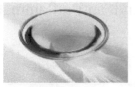 **Coconut oil, avoid cook** **78**  **Coconut Milk**	Contains the following benefits: helps lower Cholesterol level, controls Blood Sugar and Diabetes, fight Against Alzheimer's Disease, reduces High Blood Pressure, and improves Liver Health.

79 **Coconut Jelly**	Blood cleanser and promotes reproductive hormones.
80 **Olive oil, avoid cook**	Contains the high antioxidant, helps in the prevention of stroke, fight against heart disease, and helps in weight loss.
81 **Sesame oil**	It contains a rich amount of vitamins, and minerals, and antioxidants. Fight against some diseases in the body. It contains antibacterial and anti-inflammatory components.
82 **Seeds of Grape oil**	Helps moisturize skin, treat acne, skin lightening, and tighten up pores.

83

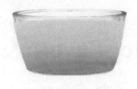

Hemp Seed oil

Decreases the danger **of** Heart Disease, helps skin health, they are plant-based protein and minimize menopausal crises.

Chapter 4

Dr. Sebi's Approved Spicy Savors & Pungent with Medicinal Benefits

Recipes	Medical Benefits
84 **Savory**	Diarrhea, sore throat, cough, nausea, gastrointestinal disorder, constipation, lack of appetite, muscular cramps, prevent dehydration and regulate the intake of water and excretion urine.
85 **Thyme**	It contains Vitamin A, Vitamin C, iron, copper, manganese and fiber Stomach pain, sore throat, arthritis, diarrhea, acne, constipation or indigestion and cold.

The Thyme Oil fight against fungal, bacteria and spasmodic.

86	Painful kidney conditions, cough, menstrual contraction, infections, cold, painful nerve and muscle, ulceration of the vaginal tract, pile/hemorrhoid, body fever, spasm, insomnia (sleeplessness), bronchi disease

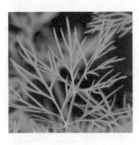

Dill

87	Controlling diabetes, detox, antibiotics, promotes healthy heart function, rapid wound recovery, suppresses inflammation, aids anti-constipation, relieves cold, coughs and other respiratory disorders, rejuvenates body tissue, etc.

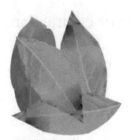

Bay Leaves

88	It cleanses the blood, anti-inflammation, relieves pains, arthritis such as osteoarthritis and rheumatoid arthritis; throat opens sore, mild fever, cough, cold, flu, headache and prevent diabetes.

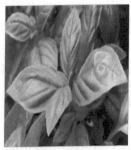

Basil & Sweet Basil

89	Correct bad appetite, tooth pain, induces moderate sleep, calm body system, emmenagogue, anti-constipation, promotes digestion, relieves muscular pain or contraction, stomachic, reduces blood sugar, diuretic,

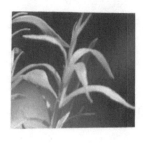

Tarragon

90	Antibiotics, anticancer, improves healthy bones, reverses high blood pressure, hinders ulcer of the

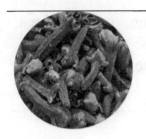 stomach, improves healthy liver, anti-inflammation, healthy function of the heart and health mouth cavity.

Cloves

 91

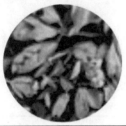 Antioxidant, anticancer, antibacterial, anti-inflammation and antivirus.

Dr. Sebi's Approved Moderate Savor with Their Medicinal Benefits

These savors are every essential in the preparation of your therapeutic diet(s) to control or reversing any health discomfort. But, the quantity should be very small in the preparation of your food, some will only require just half to one teaspoon in your food formulation because the excess may cause a burning sensation, internal heat, severer pain, inflammation, running nose, etc.

Savors	Medicinal Benefits
92 **Bird Pepper Africa**	It helps in reversing diabetes, control the level of blood sugar, protect heart, relieves stomach ache, antibiotics, and gastrointestinal disorders,
93 **Fresh Cayenne**	It controls the digestive system, regulates appetite, pain killer (analgesic), reverses high blood pressure, antioxidant, inhibits the growth of cancer and anti-inflammation.
94	It is effective for indigestion, heartburn, decreases excessive sweating and high secretion of the salivary gland,

Sage	stomachic, brain calmness, improves appetite, a retentive memory, eliminates depression, diarrhea, etc.
95 **Achiote**	It reduces fever, diabetes, improves body osmoregulation, preserves water in the body, fights malaria, antimicrobial, aids healthy liver function, purifies the body, antioxidant and anticancer.
Also, Check #54 **Pulverized Onion**	Antioxidant, anticoagulant, anticancer, antimicrobial, relief inflammation, reduces blood sugar concentration, detox, tonic, relieves migraine headache, reverse hypertension.

96	It is an antioxidant, anticancer, reverses hypertension and diabetes, removes bad cholesterol, prevents an increase in body weight and reduces fat deposit.
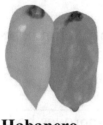**Habanero**	

Dr. Sebi's Approved Sweet Sensational Savor

Items	Medicinal Benefits
97 **Purified Cactus Agave Syrup**	Antioxidant, eliminates cancer, prevents and relieves inflammation, fight against fungal infections and bacterial infections and calms abdominal conditions.
98 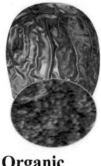 **Organic Date Sugar**	It contains fiber, zinc, potassium, iron, manganese, phosphorus, calcium, antioxidant, anticancer, controlling diabetes, reduction of blood sugar

concentration and provides sustainable

energy.

Dr. Sebi's Approved High Salt Containing Savor

These savors are inevitable in your healthy alkaline diets formulation. You only need to add an extremely small quantity of sea salt in your diets from a pitch to one-eight of a teaspoon; it is accurate to meet your sensational taste. You need to know that Sea Salt reduces high blood pressure to a normal level, but if you engage in the excess usage of it your blood pressure may result in very low blood pressure also called hypotension which very more dangerous and highly deadly than hypertension.

Therefore, consider very little quantity in your food preparation. You can take a teaspoon below from other algae powders.

Savors	Medicinal Benefits
99 **Pulverized Granulated Seaweed**	It enhances the adequate function of the alimentary canal or gut, facilitates the reduction of body weight, manages diabetes, tonic, awesome Vitamin K, iodine, iron and promotes the function of Thyroid.
100 **Purified Sea Salt**	It reverses high blood pressure, enhances the function of the heart and guides against atherosclerosis, heart disorder, partial or permanent stroke with aid of an adequate quantity of Sodium chloride

presence.

| 101 | It contains Vitamin C, zinc, manganese; performs Antioxidant, anticancer, relieves cold, cough, protects heart disorder, anti-oxidative stress |

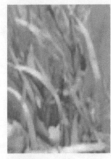

Kelp

| **Also, Check # 52** | Rich in Vitamins and Minerals. Rich in Antioxidants. It is also rich in Tyrosine, Which Supports Thyroid Function. |

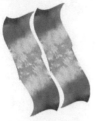

Fresh Nori

Sea

It improves gut health, decreases the risk of heart disease, and reduce weight.

Also, Check # 49

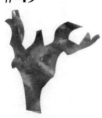

It contains calcium and potassium which helps in improving bones, reduce blood pressure, improve your eyesight and

Fresh Dulse

Sea Vegetable	improve the health of the thyroid gland.

Dr. Sebi's Medicinal Herbal Products For Alkaline Diets

The table below contains all the advisable Dr. Sebi's active ingredient of the various herbal medicines you can prepare either drinking alone or you add the extracted fluid with you diets or smoothies to facilitate rapid recovery or provide permanent body requirement for your adequate good living.

Herbal Medicine	Active Ingredient(s)	Medicinal Benefits
102	Cuachalate	To relief gastric,
Dr. Sebi	*Amphipterygium*	ache stomachaches,
Stomach	*adsstringens*	like stomach
Calming	**Dosage:**	cancer, kidney
Herbal Tea	1½ Tea should be	diseases & painful
	boiled with 2	gastric ulcer,

	cups of distilled water.	urinary pain or any disorder, mild wound & mouth diseases &
103 **Dr. Sebi\s Nerve or Stress Relief Tea**	**Chamomile** **Dosage:** 1½ Tea should be infused in 2 cups of hot water for 10 to 15minutes	It initiates relaxation and induces sleep, enhances mood, little sedative, muscular relaxation, declines irritation, everyday benefit antioxidant, controls irritable intestine syndrome, antibiotics, calm

		anti-inflammatory and stomach upset.
104 **Energy** **Booster Tea**	**Muicle** **Dosage:** 1½ Tea should be boiled with 2 cups of distilled water.	Improve your energy to the optimal healthy stage, Enhance the transportation of oxygen in your blood tissue, Antioxidant, detoxification, Blood Cleanser,
105 **Dr. Sebi's** **Immune**	**Elderberry** **Dosage:**	Prevent immune abnormality, Antioxidant.

Support Herbal Tea	1½ Tea should be infused in 2 cups of hot water for 10 to 15minutes	Prevent inflammation in mucous membranes even sinuses, exhibits fight against carcinogenic tissue of cancer and reduces cholesterol, antiviral,
106 **Dr. Sebi's Bromide Plus Powder**	**Bladderwrack** *Fucu vesiculous* **Irish Sea Moss**	Bladderwrack contains Iodine, Bromine, Mannitol, Beta-carotene, Alginic, and

Potassium.

Dosage:

1 Teaspoon to your smoothie preparation

For healthy bone and improving thyroid gland, inhibits appetite to control intestine, dysentery, pulmonary diseases, respiratory conditions, and poor breath.

For you to learn more on:

● *How to determine healthy alkaline diets formulation.*

Full knowledge about the preexisting Dr. Sebi's approved therapeutic alkaline diets and the new health-promoting formulated alkaline diets to prevent all types' diseases.

Then you will need to get my books titled:

1. Dr. Sebi Alkaline Diets Encyclopedia.
2. Dr. Sebi Approved Therapeutic Alkaline Diets.

You can also get my book for other diseases for you to learn the general healing mechanisms of Dr. Sebi using herbal medicine and some relevant complementary diets.

Dr. Sebi: Secret Methods to Detoxify Body; Cure Cancer, Kidney and Liver Diseases, Prostatitis & Be Revitalized via Dr. Sebi's Alkaline Diets & Herbs

Acknowledgment

First and foremost I appreciate the God almighty forgiven me the huge privilege to complete this health-promoting awesome *Dr.Sebi' Alkaline Diets Encyclopedia"*. Deeply, I express my profound gratitude to my wife, family for their support and more importantly the late Dr. Sebi and his family because of his tremendous humanitarianism, competency and integrity in providing hope for those who are hopeless health wisely and his evergreen life-sustaining therapeutic alkaline diets are ever living in my heart.

References

1. https//drsebicellfood.com

2. Campbell. Reece. Urray. Cain. Wasserman. Minorsky. Jackson (2008). Biology. Person Benjamin Cumming, San Francisco. Eighth Edition.

Made in United States
Troutdale, OR
11/07/2023

14387586R00054